Weird Girl with a Tumor

By

Sierra Crislip

WEIRD GIRL WITH A TUMOR

Manufactured in the United States of America
First printing October 2018

Contents

Introduction

A brain tumor is considered a serious brain injury. This story is my perspective – a version from a brain, a traumatized brain. It's my goal to share my story, so that others, too can come in and out of the darkness.

As I am writing this, I am using every piece of information I can remember. Some things I cannot even remember that have happened to me. My learning disability has taken a big toll on my life. Each and everyday I have learned to live with it and embrace it. I am going to describe what the aftereffects became like, later in the story.

"All the Small Things"

~

Blink-182

I share these stories about my childhood with trepidation. As an adult, I look back and know now that my mother was doing the best she could. However, I had a difficult time. Years later a neuropsychologist told my mother that I didn't see social situations as others do. This is my story. So my perception of how I was treated might not truly be what was happening.

Growing up, I was raised by my mom, along with my two older brothers. I was born in Pleasanton, Calif. My mother and father divorced when I was close to a year old. My brothers did the best they could to help my mom raise me.

Writing all of this helps me to overcome my past. If it weren't written, I'd be bringing it up nonstop to my family like a storm. So I am going to dive deep into my childhood and move on from there. The only way to get rid of this trauma from the past is to express it. Let me start out about my family situation.

The mystery on whether my subliminal prayers would be answered or ignored became quickly altered from dream to reality. I would have 10 seizures a day. At times, I'd try to get out of the car while on the freeway. My mom had thoughts that someone was poisoning me. This went on for nine whole years before we found a solution.

When I was five, I was diagnosed with epilepsy, with daily episodes of seizures continuing until surgery in 2004. I was born healthy and on time but was slightly slower in my early development of speech. I was behind every kid. Poor social skills were at the top of my troubles.

In my early years, my behavior was out of control, as I would have rages, be aggressive, and throw tantrums. At the same time, I was friendly, fun, sweet and compassionate. So I had many different personalities in random sequences. At one time, my aunt spent the night at our house. She slept in my room, and I was angry that I found one of her hairs on my pillow. I had a lot of empathy toward old people. They would make me cry. I'd ask my grandma if she hurt herself one time when I saw a mole on her chin. If I saw someone with a cast on at the stores, I'd ask them in a sympathetic way if they were okay. Sometimes I'd see strangers and ask my family, "Don't you love her?" or "Why don't you kiss her?" There was just this natural compassion I had for other's well-being, so it was like I was playing doctor.

Out of the blue I would laugh and hallucinate. At places, I'd randomly point and be like, "Aw, look at that girl over there?" when there was nothing there. When I was 3 or 4, my family went to the Oakland Zoo. There was some commotion and someone in the family said, "Sierra is having a seizure." My Aunt Betsy came over and saw me asleep on the ground. Another thing I totally remember was looking at the flamingo's at the zoo and calling them "pretty pink ducks"! My little brain thought ducks and birds are the same thing. I would look brain dead after I'd be passed out from seizures. It would look like I was 300 lbs. I had major Obsessive Compulsive Disorder. I collected shampoo bottles that I never even used. I would wake up my mom and tell her the visor was down in her car. Sometimes I'd let her sleep until she put it back up.

Perfectionism was at the top of my list too. Literally everything had to be exemplary. I would easily notice if something was out of place. My lip balm had to be lined up and super perfect, in straight, exact rows. My dolls all lined up on my bed, in a certain order too. Just about everyday, I always wore my pink sweats to school. One time I was on my way to school and started walking back home all angry because my sweats were in the laundry.

My family didn't know I had epilepsy until I was about 5 years old. They only saw symptoms such as laughing, seeing things that aren't there, passing out, and night walking. My mother said my legs would stiffen, sometimes I would drool, and my eyes would roll back. My mother would cry. I had a hard time making friends because of my OCD.

Each day, I would have multiple seizures, including generalized tonic-clonic, complex partial, and gelastic seizures. To this day, I could only remember those periods of uncontrollable laughter. All of a sudden, I'd get random bursts of energy and then clunk out right after. I could not stop my laugh while these episodes of seizures were going on. As a child, I remember the laughing Elmo was my favorite toy. I would say that's how my seizures have felt was like Elmo. Just press and the tickling sensation began.

My family and I have faced hardships and tried its best to find a solution. My social skills were natural, and I was good at being bubbly. I'd say whatever came to my mind. I could remember getting coached on tons of thing's I'd say. Growing up in the neighborhood, I knew just about every person in each household and would easily be friends with them all. I always said hello to anyone, especially strangers. I used to go to their house and hang out with them and their pets. I remember blowing bubbles for fun.

I'd knock on everyone's door just to say hello and or to ask if the kids could play. At times, though, I could remember the parents answering the doors and kneeling down to me saying, "Shhhh, they're sleeping." They knew how excited I was to play with the kids. In fact, a neighbor that lived across from me had some developmental disability, and we clicked like best friends. We'd ride bikes together and pretend to get gas at any nearby fire hydrant. We were just being silly kids. His name was Lucas.

I remember the exact way he pronounced my name, due to his disability. He would call me something like "See wee woah woahs."

To go back to preschool, I remember when the teacher called my mom telling her that I was being mean and hitting other kids. I could definitely remember having those rage attacks and hitting kids. At times when I'd have a seizure in the middle of class, I'd lose control and rub my hands together. On the first day of kindergarten, my mother got called to the school because my teacher said I was looking out the window and not paying attention in class. The teacher called a week later and thought I was being abused. Paramedics even came to my school when I was passed out. I would look completely brain dead- and that had teachers in panic mode.

*   *   *   *   *

After my mother got called by the kindergarten teacher and a few of other "odd" behavior episodes, such as chasing a hat in the wind....when I didn't even have a hat, my mom took me to the pediatrician. He immediately ordered an EKG of my brain. When he called my mom with the results, he said there were some abnormalities and referred me to a Local Children's Hospital.

A misfiring of the brain, they told my mom.

After that, there were numerous medications that always had to change because my seizures would break through.

I was this weird girl in those years. The other kid's had no idea what was happening to me.

I had to do first grade all over again. I didn't understand at all. I would have a seizure and then pass out. I would usually pee my pants, so the other kids made fun of me. Once you are "That Kid," it is hard to not be anymore.

My mom got in fights with one teacher who, afraid I would fall, wouldn't let me play on monkey bars at recess. My mom wanted me to be treated like a normal kid. The school would call my mom and tell her to pick me up. She would let them know that I had a right to a public education like anyone else. Finally, I had a compassionate teacher that brought in a bean bag chair and would have me rest after a seizure – all the kids in that class knew and were nicer.

This was eight entire years of that tumor growing inside my brain like a weed. No one could see it mentally or physically, of course. My family was still looking for answers on a daily basis. I looked normal just like every other kid. Seizures, as far as I can remember, felt like a tickle of lightning. I remember they made me alert, but afterward fatigue would come right after.

My physical appearance was absent of any abnormalities. I learned how to swim at such a young age, like a pro. However, I always was supervised in case seizures would occur. My brother had to jump into the pool to get me one time when I almost drowned. I remember learning to ride my bike when I was in kindergarten. It wasn't for long that I needed training wheels. Through first and second grades, I rode it to school everyday and parked it in the same spot. I wasn't really knowledgeable on how to lock up my bike, but I remember bringing the lock with me and just placing it on my tire.

My Hypothalamic Hamartoma was still unknown. As far as I can remember, I'd have gelastic, laughing seizures throughout the entire day and sometimes even during the night. I'd pass out usually a couple minutes after a seizure. Sometimes, I'd sleep walk into the streets? The uncontrollable laughter I'd face with my seizures came whenever an episode would come on, it is hard to describe what seizures felt like. I would usually describe it was a brain tickle because the moment I'd feel it go on, I'd laugh. My academic levels were below average. My seizures made keeping up in first grade difficult. Therefore, I was held back as there was an overload of work I had missed out on.

A terrifying moment was when I was found sleeping in the middle of the field during a school carnival at my school. I can recall that I would be hyper and run all over the place in a flash. I disappeared from my brothers, and it wasn't until after the carnival that they had found me.

Sometimes when my mom would go to the bank,

I'd be passed out on the floor by her shoe. During car rides after I'd have a seizure, I would always be passed out and wake up on one of my brother's shoulders. I could not even recall the moment I fell asleep.

Numerous trips to doctors and pediatricians were made to find the answer to what was going on with me. My mother at the time, worked for a neurologist who recommended we go to University of California San Francisco for a pet scan. They had discovered my tumor after the PET scan was performed. I was in need of a specialized surgery for my situation. This one doctor performed an EEG on my brain. He then called my mom to inform her there were off rhythms. We then got sent to Children's Hospital in Oakland. Whenever I'd see the BART train go by, I'd yell "I'm going off the rails on a crazy train!" I loved that song so much. It proved to be that song was my life story at the time. The pediatrician informed my mom that I had epilepsy. She had a beautiful Australian accent that I'll always remember.

Not too long after I was through with second grade, my mom, brothers and I had moved to Lathrop, California. I made friends with the neighbors in our new neighborhood. There were plenty of times that I'd get picked on by them or hated on. As always, I'd get away from the house and hang out with my friends. My tumor was still in my head, so that is probably what has helped me make friends. It wasn't going to be too long though that it would be staying inside my brain. The clock was ticking.

"Time of Your Life"

~

Green Day

My uncle did some research and found the Hope for Hypothalamic Hamartoma Foundation the same day I was diagnosed. He mentioned that the doctor located in Australia has trained the doctor in Arizona, who we ended up going to.

This is where the plan was turning into some action. The year was 2004. I was eight at the time, but turning nine pretty quick. I had barely started third grade. It was August, so I missed a couple weeks of school to go to Arizona. Prior to the Arizona trip, my uncle's church laid their hands on me and blessed me with Holy Water. I could remember looking at everyone sitting in the room watching. I had this little grin on my face. A nice lady there at the church generously gave me a Precious Moment's Bible with a unique cover! I had always kept in on my bookshelf. The last seizure I had was on the way to the airport to go to Phoenix for my surgery. I missed my first airplane ride, since I was passed out from a seizure. We caught another plane and were about to enjoy some leisure time away from California. Through my mom's love for exploration, I started to acquire some love for traveling. This was my first time going on a plane. Lot's of other family members wanted to come, but my mom weaned them from coming. She was in distraught with my surgery. The place we stayed at was in Scottsdale on a golf course.

Moments were captured as my photographer brother filming special moments throughout the Arizona trip. The background music was "Time of Your Life" by Green Day. Throughout the trip, I can remember him having me on camera in the car, and I said in a sad voice, "Oh hi, welcome to Phoenix."

My mom and I embraced the warm weather so much. We have always been into chilling out and swimming. I remember pictures being taken and we had a nice dark tan from the Arizona hot.

My surgery took place just days before my ninth birthday. I felt brave the night before. I asked my mom if they were going to take my head apart like the mannequins at Mervyns. Thankfully, once the tumor was removed, I've been seizure-free.

When I woke up from my surgery, I asked for McDonalds. My brother was filming when I asked for it. In recovery, I watched *Toy Story 2* over and over. There was an OCD I had with this movie and soon memorized each line. My mother was actually right beside me when I woke up that morning, and what a great blessing it was for the doctors to let her be right there with me through this huge surgery. They let her stay the night.

I sure did not want to leave Arizona. It felt like a dream home/vacation just being there. I remember looking through the windows on the plane at the clouds. It was nice to end the Arizona trip with my birthday. It was so much fun and will always remain a memory.

I can recall a couple of other times that my mom and I flew to Arizona to follow-up. One was in May 2006 when I was in fifth grade. We were there for just about a day and a half. I remember playing brain games. Even though I had anxiety going to the doctors, I sure didn't have anxiety flying out of California. I was especially excited to miss a day of school. Flying and traveling take away my anxiety in a flash. My mom and I didn't rent a car. We would just walk wherever we had to go. Everything was within walking distance.

Another time that we flew to Arizona was summer 2013 for a neuropsychological evaluation. This trip was going to feel like leisure time. I have seen a variety of doctors there, such as an endocrinologist, psychiatrists, and even a nurse friend we saw last time.

We were there for a week. A medical report was made. The purpose was to document my current neuropsychological status and to make recommendations for my clinical care. After doing tests, my memory was scored pretty low. This was the same as attention and executive functions.

I was amazed at all these facts and my history.

It was like reading an autobiography. All the testing was was boring, and I had a difficult time remaining on task. My significant worry and anxiety have played some roles in these academic challenges. At the end of my report, the diagnostic impressions were listed as Anxiety Disorder, Cognitive Disorder, and a Behavior Disorder secondary to Hypothalamic Hamartoma.

"Breakaway"

~

Kelly Clarkson

Things have gone downhill just a bit when we returned to California from Arizona. It was the beginning of darkness starting to follow me. I had to, unfortunately, switch to a new school, as my current school was "full." On my first day back, I was in the third grade. I felt so lost, nervous, scared and didn't even feel the same as I was before with a tumor in my head. I had absolutely no social skills at all. Actually, I wasn't skilled in anything. It felt like a part of me was missing. I was wandering through a dark tunnel. I was this different girl. For sure I was a different human, inside and outside without a tumor. All of a sudden, I was like a car that wouldn't run because of a dead battery.

I became a victim of bullying. Not one day would go by where I wouldn't get bullied. Feelings of sadness and tension were sky high. I'd get dirty looks from a few of the kids. This had me becoming afraid and shaky. I wondered, "What did I do wrong? Why don't they like me?" I remember appearing timid, scared and tense. I felt so terrible and ugly that no one liked me. During the time while this was happening, though, I just dealt with it every day and faced it.

My mom has said that I seemed more insecure after the surgery. The tumor wasn't necessarily my best friend, but it felt I had lost my best friend with the start of the bullying. Everything just turned upside down. It has never felt the same.

Kids made negative assumptions of me such as stuck up, weird and snooty. I didn't have even one friend. My school picture was even made fun of.

With my learning disability and months of struggling to keep my grades up in third grade, I got put into Special Ed for the rest of my time in school. It was a lot easier for me, and the pace felt more at my regular pace The student's silliness would pester me to the point where I'd complain and request for the teachers to make everyone be quiet.

Due to me having trouble making friends and poor social skills, I also requested at lunchtime back in elementary school to eat lunch in the office. It was the only place I could feel relaxed and at ease. I remember when being served lunch by a student she'd rip just a portion off the pizza to give to me. Better yet, I told on her and she got talked to I knew in my head that she was bullying me in a sneaky way. Everyone took they're time out of lunch just to tease and humiliate me until I'd get out the door. They wouldn't even eat their lunch with me just sitting there. I was treated like a fly they were trying to kill.

Trying to just find a seat in the cafeteria took almost my whole lunch. I always peaked at the clock in the office at my lunch and ate slowly so I'd be done close to class time. I didn't want to have to expose myself and be seen by the bullies. The risk of going to recess was threatening to me. I just could not handle any pressure or worry about being in the spotlight. I hated being the center of everyone's attention. Lunch was not a time that I could waste on and miss out on my fuel.

There was no time to even feel that sense of confidence. I always worried about what would go wrong rather then right. I constantly stumbled every time I walked and so feared people staring at me. Tension in my shoulders would occur. My talking was a constant stutter. My voice would get hoarse. I'd have to cough a hundred times. This went on everyday, from class to class, and even at the after school program. During the afterschool program, I was a volunteer, being the oldest of most kid's. It was hard and scary for me to be brave near the little kids. It was part of my duty to help them with homework. Worse case, I couldn't even understand how to do their homework. This gave them a reason to bully me.

Kids would always tattle on me for not smiling, talking or just anything "little." It was all the small things. I'll admit that I would usually mug people who stared at me because I honestly would fear they were talking about me. It was the way I responded to stress and anxiety. I was hitting puberty early around this time. I remember getting really bad stomach aches during class and had no clue why I was having them. Despite my painful stomach aches, I didn't want to go home. I chose to suffer and stay caught up in my work. In 2005, we moved to Manteca from Lathrop. I was just starting fourth grade. The thought of going to a new school again and possibly meeting other bullies just didn't seem like a decision to me. I just wanted to go with the same routine everyday and not make any small or big changes. This took a lot of time through the morning, but we made it work out. It was just a 10-13 minute drive. I didn't like changes at all. Moving to a different house and city was enough of a major change.

My mom had to drop me off at the donut shop every morning before school, because she had to rush to work. It was just a few blocks away from my school. School didn't start until late morning, 9 a.m. It was quite a dysfunctional time. There were not many other places to take me.

I had no worries of being late. At the donut shop, I got to know the owners and bought a donut almost each morning. This routine went on for about a school year. They had a son who was in my special ed class. He was a nice kid to me. My eye was always on the clock. At 15 minutes before school starting, I'd get up and walk to school through the neighborhood, rain or shine.

A couple of challenging but worthwhile moments happened in fifth grade was Science Camp and getting

100% on a U.S. states capitals test. I was the only one in class who got it all right! I was so indecisive about going to Science Camp. Constant overthinking and worry about the other kids and being away from home had me in apprehension mode. My teacher gave me some heads up on what it was like at Science Camp, though, and I decided to just go.

I felt insecure around the other girls in my cabin, as I drew attention to myself with my quietness. They stopped what they were doing just to put my quietness on the spot. I put my head down and felt humiliated. Every time we'd have a little recess time at Science Camp, I'd just find a place to sit and put my head down. My mom and I emailed from the teacher's computer. At night, I remember opening my eyes to the sound of rain outside. There were some nights I could not sleep. I remember every morning going into the cafeteria and sitting with the group of people we were picked to be with. The other kid's that were in my group were always laughing and bothering me. The ride home from science camp, I remember we passed by the theater in my grandma and grandpa's town. I had feelings that I wish I would be there. Boy, was I happy when we got back to town to return home, just to be with my family. Still, at least I experienced what Science Camp was like. I took a big chance at fear.

When sixth grade came along, I was getting on my last nerve with all of the bullies. At the start of each morning, I'd be in mainstream class with my special ed classmates. The bullying went on like a vacuum. I got suspended for standing up to a bully. This was gut-wrenching!

Coming back to school the next day, I got constantly bothered by the kids. They acted like dumb idiots. Pounds of stress and anxiety grew inside of me and it was hoping to explode. The kids were so annoying and just always finding easy ways to make me mad. The bullies were able to get away with anything, and getting me in the spot. The teachers hardly ever stood up for me.

I mostly hung out with yard duties and chitchatted with them. I felt a yearning to be with them. They had to push me away so they could do their job. This put more attention on me at recess than to the bullies. My anxiety would escalate quickly. When bullies would see me alone, I just could not show them that I didn't care, because I did, way too much.

I didn't have a problem with being a loner, the problem was with the kids teasing my about it that brought anxiety. So of course, it bothered me and I let it happen. If I started walking around, they'd just watch me more like a movie. There was no way to escape this. This journey of getting through school and dealing with bullying 24/7 was not a bit easy. Through all this tension, worry and stress, I persevered and never held back from finishing the school year. Constant feelings of apprehension and depression were controlling me, and I could feel it inside of me. I didn't have anyone trusted to talk to about school and troubles I was having. I did not have a chance to rock the boat. The pain and bitterness went through this whole journey with me everyday. Throughout the years, I have had trouble forgetting and putting the past behind. It would always run in my head like a windmill. No matter what I would be doing, the past just could never escape my head. Over time, I have tried to treat the past like taking the trash outside because you get rid of it that way. It does not need to define my future. I have learned to let it make me stronger and create a more sustainable future.

"The Middle"
~
Jimmy Eat World

In August 2009, I started eighth grade and a new school. It felt really lonesome everyday. The school wasn't even within walking distance. This new life turned my world even more upside down. The road we lived on was so busy and miles long. Luckily, the bus would pick my neighbor and I up. We would wait outside together. We were usually the first few people to get on the bus before the crowd's came along. I'd "hide" by wearing sunglasses all the time.

Hiding behind my sunglasses ironically put more attention on me by other students. So many kids teased me for wearing them. It was my hiding spot from anxiety. I thought it would drag attention away from me. If anyone looked at me in the eyes, I'd feel agitation and shakiness. Every bad habit I had of dealing with my anxiety was a big no. Sadly, my neighbor noticed them on me too. I was doing this to make people not stare at me so much because it was my biggest fear when people stared.

The first day of eighth grade was mediocre. It started out with my normal Special Ed main class.

I made friends with this girl. She wasn't my friend for very long. She eventually bullied me as well. I have changed the name of some bullies – not to protect them but to protect myself. We talked super easily and hung out a lot. She was the only "friend" I had that I got to take for my birthday dinner. At the time, I let her rule me no matter how she treated me. Just having that person by me was all I asked for. I even got to spend the night at her house. This was the only time she treated me like a real, true friend. Throughout the year, she was becoming a bully but in disguise. It turns out that she was two-faced.

The teachers treated her like a perfect teacher's pet. She was ruling me for a long time throughout school. I felt this attachment to her for some reason, as I am used to clinging to others. This was just putting negativity on myself and not positivity.

A big struggle for me back then was to focus. I was powerless more than ever. Whenever I'd get home after school, I'd go straight into my room. I'd read a book, or even draw rock band logos. Most nights, I remember I would write in my journal to talk about the day. I remember the start of my journal usually stating "Today was a bad day." Probably only 1% of the time it was a good day. This was my creative mindset when I was bored. Just going to my room and being stranded in there was how I dealt with it. I hardly went to any social events, especially with kid's my age. By the end of each school day, I was feeling drained from all the action at school. The only way I found myself a little braver at school would be when bullies were absent.

On a positive note, during a marathon in eighth grade, I ran the most laps out of everyone in my grade. Therefore, I won the race and earned a delicious In-N-Out lunch with the principal along with student winners from other grades.

Out of everyone in my special ed class, I was the only one who was put in mainstream classes, which were history and science. I felt intimidated by the kids, as they were also bullies and smarter then me. After months went by, I had my mom request that I get out of the class. It was so much pressure and anxiety for me. My mind was always boiling like hot water every morning that I walked into that class. Eventually I didn't have to go to that class anymore. The teacher was shocked that I wanted out. She was enjoying me in that class, but I backed out.

The school photographer captured a family pic of my parents, brother, grandma and me. It was just the middle of my journey being almost over. It was only "The Middle" that just took some time.

I was sure looking forward to a long nice summer at my favorite places. It was either my maternal grandpa's or my paternal grandma's. They were fun to be around, and I loved all the laughs we'd share.

I wouldn't trade any time to be with my grandparents. We always had special bonds. I visited them both whenever I'd be in town. They were just about less then a mile away. Every moment spent with them was enjoyed. I remember going out to breakfast a lot with my grandpa and running errands for him, or washing his dishes. My grandma was my main go-to buddy. We'd have endless conversations, and I'd never get anxiety speaking to her.

It would get dreading when summer would come to an end, and I'd have to go back home and get ready for school and all the negativity and harassment. I was doing the things that I love rather then being surrounded by negativity. It was more peaceful to be surrounded by loving people than hateful, negative kids. There was no better summer then spending it with my grandma or grandpa.

"The Climb"

~

Miley Cyrus

Around August 2010, a new anxiety chapter began. Being a victim of bullying was continuing and never-ending. On the first day of high school with new people and new classes, oh my goodness, the anxiety and overwhelming episodes were sky high. My mother was with me, just for a short moment. She was showing me where each of my classes were, and I just felt nauseous. This painful knot was hurting inside my tummy just about every single day. However, I kept that feeling internally and let the pain keep coming. My anxiety took over, and it was going to lead me. I was in the darkest part of the tunnel.

All I could feel was anxiety and darkness ahead. The crowd of so many people felt like a baseball game to me and was driving me crazy. Crowds were my biggest nightmare and a struggle to get used to. I only felt comfortable with my mom there. I've always had that attachment problem with her. She's had to tell a doctor that I nag on her and that it bothered her.

Yet, I just went along with the flow to each class,

one at a time. I felt so intimidated by other students. I would say the kids all seemed the same as they were in elementary and middle school – immature. It was the start of just another tough roadblock. As mentioned before, my skills were still poor, no self- confidence, and it still felt like I was wandering through the dark tunnel. Freshmen year was a pretty embarrassing start for me. I had some hard classes like Home Economics. My learning disability and anxiety were my control freaks. I remember in Home Economics when we had to sew a button for a project, I was the only one who failed – good grief. I had to start all over on it. Getting behind and keeping up was tough in this class. Shortly, however, I got out of that class and switched to Child Development. It was much easier to learn and more interesting. We did a project by taking home a fake baby. I had to do it twice, as the first try for me, I took home the wrong monitor. I asked to redo the project for a passing grade.

In the locker room, I get teased at 24/7 whenever we were changing. The bathroom stalls were always taken, so I couldn't go in there. The girl's drove me insane with their bitter behavior. Even more embarrassing, I didn't even know how to use a locker on the first day. After a few tries, I got it down.

There was always something small that someone had to point out to me. Once I had my car to drive to school, people took advantage of me and started to be nice. This was only when they needed rides from me. I would take that into consideration and do what they'd all ask me to do – drive them from place to place, without asking for gas money. Honestly, I could've rejected them, but if they were nice, I just took any chance I got to have "friends" when they'd be nice. Therefore, that's why I was an easy target.

Anything the bullies would ask from me, they knew I wouldn't deny them. I was not a wise thinker. I had no clue what I was getting into. It was like a déjà vu moment. Later, I made everyone give me gas money if they needed rides. At that point, they no longer were "friends!" They were just using me. When I had to deny some of these people about rides, they automatically would cut me off and not speak to me anymore. Speaking up for myself and knowing when to say "No" was one of the hardest struggles for me. It would be an automatic loss of those bullies being "nice" to me.

As usual, I was always slow at making quick decisions. So standing up to bullies was not easy, at all. I'd gaze into space and just "think." My school ID photo haunted me the rest of the year. Throughout the year as my hair grew and kids or teachers saw my ID, it was so awkward for them to see that photo of a different me. I always had it facing backward to not let it get to me. But it actually was getting to me, since I put it backward.

This was not easy though. It brought more attention for the bullies to see me if they saw me alone. That's all the advice I'd hear from counselors and adults throughout high school. They did not understand my troubled and stressful endeavors.

Speaking of counselors, whenever I'd try to talk to them about bullies, they'd just take it lightly and say that it's okay. Oh, but when bullies would tell on me for just giving them a dirty look, the counselors would get on my behind like tailgaters. They were not very caring about me.

The biggest problem with myself was worrying too much what people thought, and letting them take control of me. Overthinking and constant worrying ran through my head like a marathon. Looking back, I did give people dirty looks and would mug them with my eyes being squinty. It was the only way I'd get in my comfortable state.

Of course, at the time I was not aware that I was giving others that impression. Never was a smile on my face. I just couldn't figure out though why no one liked me. There was just no way to get them out of my head. Not one adult in my life has understood how hurt my school experience was. Everyone wanted to only hear the "good" parts about my school – which apparently was nothing. It ruled my entire life in school.

I could not feel or appear relaxed in school ever. Shoulders clenched, rapid heartbeats, stuttering, and head down were my appearance everyday. I have learned from it, though, and am learning to just embrace who I am and not regret it. I mean I have grown out of certain characteristics I used to have but would not change my interests or introverted ways for the bullies.

At one time in high school, I had to take this van with other kids who had developmental disabilities. When it dropped us off at school, this would draw the bullies' attention to me. Heart palpitations, panic attacks, and worry would skyrocket when this happened. It felt like I was putting on a show to the bullies to find more ways to pick on me. I feared for my life. With the other rider students having obvious physical disabilities, my worrying thoughts were that the bullies would be thinking I had it too. There was no way to put this worry behind.

I made friends with the kids who rode with me, but not for long. Eventually they chose to pick on me and not be true friends.

When I'd be riding it in, I remember hiding a book in front of my face so other kids wouldn't see me in it. One kid in my PE class let the cat out of the bag and asked me, "Why do you take that van?" Uh oh, I felt like I was in hot water.

How the heck was I supposed to answer him? Adrenaline and a quick heartache would rush with a flustered face. Nothing was easy to just simply tell people without worry and fear. I was on the edge of just crying in tears. Obviously he asked me this question so he could try and call me "mental." I knew he was just trying to make me sound mental.

There was not one moment in high school where I felt relaxed, brave or stress-free. The same old cliché was said to me everyday from the kids.

So many "friends" have done this to me. I've made friends with a boy in a wheelchair who had his unique disabilities and would love being his friend. When these bullies made fun of my pimples on my face, he joined along with them and asked me, "Why do you have dots?" Later on, I stopped being his friend. If a person couldn't act like a friend to me in front of the bullies, I would be done with them. They were not true friends. But, sad to say, anytime I'd have a "friend" no matter if they were nice to me for even a hot minute, I would just go along with that and not try to confront them. As you can see, I was weak and naïve.

I tried joining the swim team, and the moment the tryouts were happening, I backed out. I was scared for my life with bullies being on the team. I was not into any social events at school no matter how exciting they'd seem, whether it was football games, homecoming, etc. Fear was my best friend. I would always dream of realistic things, but by the time they required action, that's when I'd back down.

Anything "social" was not on my interest list ever. My mom was never really shy and she always wanted me to put myself out there and make friends but she did not understand how hard it was for me. I didn't take her advice. I never talked with her closely about how awful school was. I would only vent about it to my grandma – because she would listen and not complain. I couldn't even talk to my dad about it – it would get him stirred up and overwhelmed.

At first I'd think positive, that "I got this," but my heart raced so fast that it told me no, not right now. Nevertheless, I always took trips to the local gym in town and would swim laps by myself on sunny days. It was more of my forte. No one was there to bother or bully me. I was already on a bowling league through the city and was doing well enough with just that sport.

My mom was always there to watch me, which felt like security. Sometimes my grandpa or dad would watch me at times too. My coach always tried to teach me and show me how to throw the ball, but I still kept throwing it my own style.

On a daily basis, students always told me "You look high, stoned." This really hurt my feelings so bad. I had no clue what that even meant. Thinking of the word "high" to me meant like the sky. I started doing online research at these words and was horrified with the meanings. Thank you to Urban Dictionary. Some people even said my eyes looked skimpy. I don't know why I let it bother me, but it did. I'm proud of the fact I have never done drugs or used alcohol. There was just always something they'd find to judge me about.

Electives I chose to take through high school were Art. I like art and would consider myself creative. . When I took art in sophomore year, I'd always get criticized for my artwork. I, of course, couldn't say anything right off the bat. It really hurt me so bad. In 11th grade, I took art again, and it was much better. I made a friend. She was quite like me so we clicked automatically. She made me feel so comfortable in class and not scared as much.

Having her for a nice friend was the best part of class. Out of all the bullies in school, she has never bullied or treated me bad. So luckily, I found at least one nice friend at school. Her two brothers happened to know my big brother.

I got to focus on my artwork and have those quiet moments. One of my artwork even got to be hung up in the school office. Being artistic was one of my strengths.

My kind of fun was doing normal things like eating, reading, going to the gym. I was far off from enjoying social gatherings, parties, dances, etc. In PE, I always was the one that had no "partner." I would have to beg my teacher for one, which was so uncomfortable and embarrassing to me. Sometimes I would get lucky and have one, but they'd all move on from me. In 10th grade, I requested a switch in PE classes. It was simple and worked out. I would say I liked my new PE class better then the previous one. The majority of the time I was able to have a partner in the new class. This was my biggest wish for the new PE class.

Everyday in class, I would always think in my head that one day I wouldn't have to deal with them anymore.

With the tumor not in my head anymore, it totally felt like something was missing from myself. To make this sound understandable, it's like the tumor was a fully charged battery with a ton of energy. Without it, the battery was dead and low.

Two high school teachers of mine had to talk to me once about the expressions on my face. They thought I gave them a dirty look. It's like this mean mug face put me in my comfort zone to bullies. I apologized to the teachers and said the sun was in my face. With anyone looking at me for even a minute, I just couldn't keep a calm straight face. I was feeling my way through the darkness.

I was having super high anxiety and social anxiety, panic disorder.

There was hardly ever a happy day for me at school. Each day was dark and depressing. To make it a little fun, I'd always head on over to this delicious Mexican restaurant like literally everyday after school. It was my escape route. I didn't care or worry about my weight much and the pounds would go up.

Looking back at why I did that, I think it helped me clear my head from all the tension at school so I had something to feel good about. Ironically, though, I had no self-confidence or any feeling of sureness of myself. So the bad food was like an excuse for my insecurities.

Eleventh grade was the year I was pampered for

early graduation). Thank goodness it was going to be a quick and last year with the bullies. I know that this tension wasn't going to go on forever, but it sure felt like forever while I was living in it.

Looking back, I don't know how I was able to put the bullies and my anxiety behind. I just did it and let this tension with bullies haunt me. Somehow, my anxiety was used as a powerful motivating force. My depression and anxiety were just piling up each day. All this bullying and drama every single day was one of the big reasons I wanted to graduate early and be done. You can rely on me as the "Early Bird." I always had that OCD to arrive early.

When I started driving in high school, I'd always get there 30-40 minutes early to get that same parking spot. Boy, it would get packed easy. That extra "spare" time would give me some "me" time to relax before the big long day of school. It was not a problem to me, as it assured that I got to school early and didn't have to worry about being late.

Throughout high school, I took every chance I got to hide in the bathroom at lunch. I didn't have time to go through all that trouble of trying to make friends, sit with bullies, etc. When I'd go into the cafeteria, people would throw food at me and wouldn't let me sit with them. The adrenaline would blow up like a tire and almost explode. I liked that alone time. A teacher finally caught on to where I was hiding at lunch and told me I couldn't be in the bathroom anymore. She eventually told my history teacher, who brought it up to me in front of the whole class. Then I wondered where I could find another place to eat my lunch away from the bullies. I eventually started eating in my car. I had no words and even found it sometimes hard to breathe. Being in the middle of crowds or social gatherings would drain my battery.

Going from class to class, hour after hour, was super draining for me and my head pounding would go on and on. It would be so hard to catch my breath. Anytime there'd be parties or fun gatherings in class or school, my first thoughts were like, "Please, be quiet!" I could not sense the same fun that kids and teachers had. It was tiring and just wasn't interesting to me. I'd ask teachers to please keep it quiet, and they'd get defensive with me. This one teacher told me that we are here to have fun, and if I don't have fun, to go put my head on my desk. I felt so terrible for not feeling excitement and joy in these activities.

I was just another human being, but had different perspectives and skills then the others. A therapist told my mother once that I don't see social situations like others do. I didn't really notice it when I was in school, but the feeling and thought of just "people" especially teenagers, gave me headaches or moments of sighs.

In my junior year, I had finally come to the point where I was absolutely ready, determined and all prepared to graduate "early" and get away from all those bullies. Yes, my anxiety was driving me to get to that destination. I did what it took to get my diploma months early. My head was high in the clouds and gave me a sense of power and revenge for the bullies. Getting ahead of them was my biggest wish. I spoke to a counselor and asked her what can I do to graduate early. She showed me a short list of courses I would have to take and that I'd be all set to graduate early.

My junior year seemed to flew by fast. With all that determination in my head, things didn't get to me so much. Senior year was the best of my life because I didn't have to go to high school in person and stress through all the bullies.

I actually completed my senior through an online school. I didn't completely isolate myself from everyone. Instead, I actually met inspirational, helpful teachers who helped me through this all.

My mother and I had our first meeting with a counselor at the new school, and I was so eager, telling him how excited I was to be graduating. It was August. He put out his hand out and said, "Don't put the cart before the horse." I just smiled, and we proceeded with our meeting.

My mom and I also scheduled my own senior pictures just for fun. I loved pictures and capturing moments. We took the ones with the graduation dress on and then later in the day, I got dressed up professionally and had pictures taken by a creek. I always will remember this fun day with my mom and the photographer. It was a one-on-one session.

This school felt like home to me. The teachers were very welcoming. My teacher/coordinator and I developed a close friendship and rapport together. She was very helpful and always helped me put my goals into action. The courses that I had to complete for graduation were short and simple. It was relaxing for me to do at home without much help.

A tense but worthy requirement for graduation was community service. This got me feeling a little overwhelmed, but I didn't hold back and completed it in a short few months. Soon, I was doing my best at improving my social skills.

As soon as my community service hours were all completed, I had another anxiety-provoking job to do before graduation. It was a slideshow presentation. Each day I practiced the slideshows with my teacher and kept trying until I said it with confidence. I shed tears before the big day when I had to present it to about six people, including my mom. Once in the middle of it, my voice cracked. I got back up and finished it. I was shaking and bright red. I took a deep breath and paused for a short moment then jumped back in to my presentation.

After the presentation was over and everyone gave a round of applause, I felt relieved for it to be over.

Now the graduation was getting closer. Grateful and thankful, I graduated and got my high school diploma in December 2013. That euphoric feeling was screaming in my heart going "You Did It." I was beyond excited and ready to pick up that diploma the day they called. Hallelujah! Again, the feeling of getting ahead of those bullies and graduating before them, shows them how determined people like me can get AHEAD of them. It was like the best day of my life. I could not of been happier then getting just ahead of those bullies. This was another moment of capturing photos. My photographer brother took the photos of my parents and I. Moments like this you just can't miss out on for the camera.

So in a way, it's like I'm the Class of '13 and the bullies are still a year behind me. Graduating high school early was the best way to get over the dreading bully years of school. I didn't have to go to the school and brag to them about it. I just had to focus on myself and do what it took to make it

My teacher even got me signed up for a local community college. I was of course, beyond excited, to even start. It was perfect timing too, since I was going to attend the Spring 2014 semester.

I went a little too far ahead of myself when going to college. I was so spontaneous and had many different ideas and just kept going without really "thinking."

So to speak, I randomly thought of respiratory therapy to study. I was thinking "BIG." When my mom and I spoke to a counselor about the courses to be taken for RT, oh that just made me scratch my head and not really want to do it. I had no clue I'd have to take chemistry, science, biology, math and all those complex courses.

I started out slow with some prerequisites, but dropped out after just one semester. I was not mentally prepared or ready for this challenging college life.

One memory of the college was that I got to go to prom. It was actually my first prom ever. I never got asked in high school. That's all I want to remember about college. I was quiet as always, even with the college kids. They college kid's were just more accepting of me and I tried my best to keep up their social interactions.

You see, going to college for the first time wasn't that easy. I did what was best for myself at the time and backed away. My social skills were still poor. I was indecisive and not prepared for college as I was NOT 100% sure on what I wanted to pursue my career in. After a short break, I tried again by taking business management courses and it proved to me the point that I was NOT taking my choices with enough consideration. Instead of thinking carefully, I was spontaneous and took anything for no legitimate reason. These mistakes were leading me nowhere but did follow the same old patterns. The best decision I had to make was to quit for the moment and put college aside.

"Demons"

~

Imagine Dragons

Many different routes were taken to try and treat my social anxiety. The side effects of many medications just would torture me with even more anxiety. So I didn't see why it would be a good idea to try any. I sure would not want medication to be the complete answer for my anxiety. I've tried group therapy but was adverse to it due to my social anxiety.

My anxiety would skyrocket in these situations. I even tried quite a few medications and gave them time. When the psychiatrists would tell me, "You may feel worse before you feel better," that was a complete failure. They made my anxiety much worse. I'd get more agitated, sleepy, lose my appetite, and things would get abnormal. I gave the medication's plenty of time to try and work, but my symptoms of anxiety were getting much worse then they were without medication.

Through the years, I found natural ways to help my anxiety, which were more effective. No chemistry or medications are necessary to be involved. Going on walks and exercising has been proven to help my anxiety a lot. If my mind has been filled with negative thoughts, I can get moving to walk it off. Looking back through the years, I can see that I have improved significantly on my anxiety. Over the years, I found that living with anxiety was helpful and of course, normal.

It has gotten better then before. I will live with it though for a long time and that is normal. My anxiety is like a light switch that goes on and off.

Another time, my mom and I saw a San Francisco neuropsychologist in September 2015. I found this doctor visit to be helpful and more accurate because I had more diagnoses, such as Social Anxiety and Agoraphobia. With these particular diagnoses, it seemed that I was getting to know myself even more. In fact, each detail my mom was describing about my seizures and tumor was amazing me at her memory while raising me. I had my eye on her about everything she would say.

So it's no surprise that I have agoraphobia. However, I faced this fear during my internship and went with the flow by riding it every morning. It was just a little too much driving. The anxiety I had on BART was enough to deal with. I'm glad that BART is not the only way to get places. Taking my car over public transit would be my first and foremost choice. Not being in crowds is how I would my energy back. It also helps me focus, where I have no interruptions or distractions.

"Breaking the Habit"
~
Linkin Park

During my early twenties, I have developed staggering habits such as eating disorder, weight loss, overexercising, and way more obsessed with my body image/weight. It may have been too obsessive, but in positive ways, I found that these habits have helped me to become more organized, stay on track, and remain more attentive. As I matured, I wanted to look my super best and aware of what foods I'd have. Despite a psychiatrist telling me that sweetened coffee drinks would increase anxiety, I didn't let that stop. I had to do something nice for myself and my constant worry and fear. Each and every day, I'd stop by the coffee shop for my sweet tea or coffee. While it may not of helped my anxiety go away, it sure got my motor running, and I find that to be essential to my everyday life. Sometimes I'd go through panic modes and felt scared to even walk in Starbucks, because of the crowds. So I started developing a habit of going to the drive-thru. When I'd be reminded that wasn't good for my social skills, I'd tell them that It was just time for a little spin in the car. Even if it was waiting in the drive-thru for a dragging amount of time, I was patient and wouldn't be in a hurry, as long as I didn't have to be anywhere. To decide if I felt like physically going inside Starbucks for my drink would depend on my anxiety. I'd leave it up to that and decide from there.

The other highly obsessive habit I've been accustomed to was walking and staying active. It would just give me a sense of relief to walk, helping me get away from anxiety or stress. Exploring and seeing things outside was interesting to me. When my love for walks began, I started doing it all alone. Eventually, the more I got to see people at the neighborhood park, I'd get into the habit of greeting them and smiling, because that's the impression they gave to me. The other people's dogs made me feel less anxiety and put a big smile on my face.

I wasn't the kind of person who would just like that morning walk to start the day. Walking became my new obsession. It was just my style and my way of coping with anxiety. Without going on walks, I'd feel like my head would just pile and pile. The walks would help with letting that all flow out through the air. Looking back my years in high school and the past, I never have enjoyed things like walks, healthy eating, appearance or anything in a dream girl's bag. Through these habit changes, I have seen quite a difference in my skin complexion too. Having a zit-free face while going through mountains of anxiety, fear and depression all throughout school was nearly impossible. It all showed up physically and was too hard to hide.

Getting past all this from high school and tension in my younger years like raising the bar. Anxiety was my greatest supporter through all of this and even if some of it was negative, it was positive in so many ways as well.

"Crazy Train"

~

Ozzy Osbourne

I have struggled keeping jobs. The reason is directly related to my brain tumor. The removal of the tumor caused brain trauma. My problems are directly related.

For a very long time, indecisiveness was my biggest trait. This entire journey of my jobs was highly associated with anxiety, mental anguish, stress and depression. Therefore, no wonder I was having a hard time keeping up with them.

I mostly worked in retail and fast food throughout my teenage years. The trauma I had from my brain tumor made it hard for me to keep up with jobs. I couldn't keep up with tasks, understand or learn anything, had poor social skills and high anxiety all along. The only thing I was good at was being on time and never be late.

I would experience panic attacks, anxiety and shortness of breath. The entire time, I'd keep my head face down and feel like a loser. I had a very hard time being social and had high anxiety. My heart would boil so high that a stomachache would come on.

I didn't know what I was doing with myself. I was just spontaneous and didn't read between the lines carefully. The merry-go-round was still going on.

I just jumped into things so quick. The manager coached me that I wasn't friendly enough either… that I could understand. I was quiet, reserved and not very attentive to the customers.

I wasn't aware of the job duties and personality traits that were necessary for the job.

Since I had "free" time, I started on a babysitting web page. It was a fun experience. Babysitting and hanging out with kids was enjoyable to gain work experience.

At times, I'd sometimes have low energy to keep these energizing kids entertained. Even the parents would complain. I'd feel like a failure when the parents would ask that I cook and do household chores, which I didn't know how to do.

This whole experience of finding my fit in life has gone on for years. I didn't reach out to people, know anyone, have friends, etc. As I mentioned, it was all a process of elimination. Time was going by, and I just had to move on. I've learned a lot of constructive lessons, and by babysitting I got to put myself out there a little, meet others and develop social skills, and gain knowledge of childcare. It was great basic skills I learned and have found them useful in my everyday life.

I felt so lost everyday and had no clue to what I would enjoy doing as a job, but I ALSO knew how to do the job. Time went on, and the job became awkward and weird. I'd get tired easily when socializing and talking for even a short time. If I was quiet for even just a minute with the teenage coworkers, they'd think of me as weird. This pattern went on with most jobs. Some coworkers would reach out to me sarcastically and say, "You look so happy." I wasn't aware at the time that I looked sad and anxious. I would take it as an insult and be supersensitive.

Another retail job I had was pretty difficult. I remember being excited to start at 4 a.m., since the store wouldn't open until like 8. That would give me some time to relax before the action with customers began. It was hard on my body to get used to it, but not for long. Constant complaints and warnings were given to me about how slow I was working. I couldn't comprehend how to look at a planogram and build a shelf. I wasn't aware that this was going to be part of my job.

Since I didn't mark my disability on the job application, no one could understand why I could not follow directions. It just was not a good fit for me. I felt left out because everyone else knew what they were doing, while I didn't. Sometimes I'd zone out and just overthink. My hours were going down each and everyday, so I informed the HR that I was leaving and felt that I wasn't being treated fairly.

When I left retail, I wanted to try out office work. It didn't require customer service, which I liked. Worse case, I got let go in a flash due to me not learning quick enough. It was enjoyable, but it was also super-detailed and took a lot of focus and concentration. My mind would always get distracted and wander. I bravely asked for help when I needed it, and soon they just got tired of helping me. It was a very tough period for me, as I had no one to talk to about this, did not have guidance to support me. While I honestly thought I would master this job, it was unfortunately a game loss. I also had a hard time explaining my struggles at work, as to them it looked like I was stirring up dirty laundry. Overthinking and worrying that they'd think, *I'm a lousy worker* was always present in my head.

Even more embarrassing would be when I'd see friends and family and they'd curiously want to ask me "How's the job going?" My answer about 99% of the time would be "I'm not there anymore!" Big sigh and just feelings of inhibition. I know just how crazy I drove everyone telling them of a new job over and over. It was the truth, though. The feeling of having to explain the whole story behind each job and why they didn't work out felt so tiring for me. It made me feel so insecure and little value.

Another thought about work was *Why would I want people seeing me work in there?* Sometimes,

I'd see family or friends of my mom's come in, and I wasn't the friendliest when this would happen. I felt like they were bothering me, as it was annoying. Sometimes I'd hide or act like I didn't know they were there.

I just kept on following the same patterns throughout the years. I didn't know what I was doing. At least I was aware that I would not be interested in the cash register. The stocker was the most suitable choice for me. It was good, as I was into organizing and sorting things. Still, people walking by me would make me feel so panicky and just tensed up. I'd be overthinking in my head what item they'd be getting ready to ask me about. I tried everyday to study the aisles and which items were there, but it hardly clicked in my head, unless the item was in the aisle I'd be standing right by, then I'd be able to direct the customers to the item immediately. The cash registers would be my last resort. On busy days when all associates would be called up front to the registers, I would feel like just running into the bathroom panting like a dog. I had a vent talk with a manager and told him in panic mode that I just cannot do it. From there on, they didn't bother with me doing it again. What a big huge relief this was after all the stress.

The moment that a customer would walk up to me, I'd feel this big tension and tightness in my chest. They'd notice my throat would appear clenched, so they'd ask me "Is your neck feeling okay?" My face froze and felt so embarrassed inside. I would just say that, "Yes it's fine." I know now that they were just making conversation. My face would just have this uncomfortably numb feeling from inside, as I would always be contemplating what they were about to say.

They even asked for a manager, and I felt so terribly sorry for the lady. I blamed my high anxiety. My anxiety caused me to speak super fast like a Minion. I'd even get feelings of fear with questions on where items were located. It'd make my head spin like a globe, because I just couldn't think of the answer at that exact second. Anytime customers would ask me where an item was, my learning disability was ruling inside my head telling me, *I do not know the answer.* There'd be no way that customer's would know I had a disability, as you can't see it physically.

Soon I went back to babysitting for an agency and did it off and on. I liked how the schedules were not set in stone, as it gave me some time to relax and gain my energy back.

If you are in a job or situation that you feel is uncomfortable, don't be afraid to speak up. I was just so scared that I'd cause trouble or put the managers in bad moods. This would not be easy for me. It just took a lot of practice and deep breaths. My advice would be to focus on the positives and how your differences could be adapted in this world. I've learned that if you hide your feelings and don't communicate them, people won't know what you are wanting. I sure wasn't afraid to tell managers or workers about my anxiety. It was obvious that I appeared anxious and tense, because anxiety shows up on the outside.

These characteristics and feelings were uncontrollable, and I could not make them go away. I've climbed mountains to work on it. Those types of job environment's are not my forte and I would not plan to be in those shoes again. There goes some thing's crossed off my grocery list. As time has been going on, I got to know myself a little more with the help of books, magazines, and anything technical.

"Best of You"

~

Foo Fighters

During November 2015, I had an opportunity that was a great move for me.

Luckily, a friend of my aunt's mentioned to her about a state resource program she worked for previously. These encouraging words from her were so motivational that I promptly followed her. She hooked me up with them fast.

I was able to meet with my case manager. I put on my brave soul because I knew I was heading on the right track to finding my fit. Without the help of my aunt's friend, I probably never would have got in touch with these helpful resources.

As our meeting went on with my case manager, she informed me of an internship opportunity through them for people with disabilities. It was like a replacement for college and sounded like a great opportunity. The part that it's for people with disabilities, gave me a sense of confidence; all of the students would all be related somehow with our differences. I signed up and was more ready then ever. It was with the County of Alameda, located in Oakland, California.

In September 2015, my mom and I had a special appointment with a doctor in San Francisco. I was tested all day. At the end of the day, the doctor told my mom and I if I had a broken leg, people would open the door for me. I had a disability, and it was in writing. My struggles are real. You just cannot see it. On going back to Phoenix – the doctors wanted us to because the tumor is so rare; they wanted me to get follow-ups to observe the long-term effects.

My OCD was to always be at the train station early enough so I could stand in line first. I always hated being between and behind people in line. It's part of my early bird characteristic. At times, when I had no choice but to be in the back of the line, the train doors would close on me, which agitated me as I had to wait for a later train. Being on time (or early) is one of my best and most important traits I have. As you can see, I am very mindful and attentive with time. It has always been on my important list.

Classmates of mine sometimes would get on the train when it stopped at some of the stations on the way to Oakland. I just did my usual and listened to my headphones. Still, though, I would prefer not to take it.

This was a year-long program. We were provided with job coaches. The way that this program worked was each student would get assigned to different worksites, 3 months at each place.

My classmates and I helped out with clerical tasks. We were not required to do any customer service type duties. I would say that has helped me be comfortable with what I was doing. Extra time to do work was a sense of relief.

Having the job coaches checking on us every now and then felt like a sense of security. We were notified that they'd be just a text or call away if we needed help. Class started around 9 a.m. every day. For that hour, we'd learn job skills and do work related activities.

Later in the program, the teacher introduced us to ergonomics. We did it the last 10 minutes of class before going to our worksites. She would conclude it by us doing a "follow your thumb" game, telling us to pick a partner. My anxiety rushed to the top, making it hard for me. I had some luck with a partner, but mostly I was alone and felt embarrassed. I had to fake my feelings to others, letting them know I'd be okay without a partner. This was a flashback to high school. I politely informed the teacher on my hardships in school and that if she would please not have us pick partners.

Our worksites sometimes would have luncheons and invite interns to stay and eat with them. I usually backed out and went straight to my classroom for my own lunch. I was already drained from being with them throughout that hour. I needed a break and some fresh air.

At the end of each rotation, we'd receive evaluations and a big thank you for working with them. I mostly got averages.

I remember how after the first rotation the work department's said it was a pleasure having me, but that I needed to be more open. They said I appeared reserved. I felt so self-conscious and awkward. Well, it was a completely new work environment for me, and I'm sure all the interns were a bit timid at first like me. I would make sure I greeted everyone, at least. Seeing them focused on their computers made me not want to interact with them because I can see they were busy.

This really confused me with my social anxiety. I got along with each employee. We had fun making conversation and working at the same time. But if there was too much talking, it cost us a talk with the supervisor. At the end of each rotation, our worksites would throw each of us little parties. I backed out of events like this, as I didn't want all the attention.

By January 2017, we were nearing the end of the program. All our resumes were getting updated. This program was 11 months long. I was offered an opportunity but was not ready for it at that moment.

They always told me I am great with people and friendly. The way I take it is that I don't consider myself a people person or social, it's just that I have grown out a little bit of my shell and have learned and practiced some useful skills. I was able to speak a little more clear and precise.

I just wasn't ready for this challenge too soon. As usual, it took me a long time to get settled with new things. "Trying" it out was just making my brain go blank. The internship was a great step to improving my social and work skills.

During the graduation ceremony, seeing my parents sitting together helped calm my anxiety a lot. Nothing could have made it any better. My heart was filled with joy.

Previous graduates spoke about their experiences. They had more visible disabilities then you would see on me. I loved hearing the stories of such amazing people. Hearing the inspiring stories of others gave me a positive reminder that even a person with physical disabilities can achieve great things. One previous graduate spoke about her struggles but did not give up and kept trying harder. I took her advice and told myself that if I take the initiative, I can do it too.

Suddenly, I was trying to always look toward the bright side and think of what I COULD do, instead of what I COULDN'T.

I tried keeping up with the job clubs that the director of the program held. It was getting too much. I started going on my own and advocating for myself. The job clubs were held every other Friday and just the thought of driving there, sitting down and listening to them speak and chat for two hours straight just exhausted me. At first, it was helpful with them teaching us job and interview skills, but It wasn't really making my confidence grow. I told myself that I would just go out and advocate for myself. I thanked them for their help.

Every time I thought I was going down a new road of better choices and jobs, I kept hitting the same roadblocks. This was going on until I stopped and thought of ways to stop repeating these things. So I tried each out for help with supportive people and fought the fear of my anxiety.

My case manager gave me some resources to try out and that would be beneficial to me. I went back to this local agency in my town and get assistance with job searching. I met a new counselor. I liked how straightforward, structured, and thorough she was.

She gave me such great motivation that I had to show perseverance. Her advice and motivation really put me in line and I needed that encouragement. Going back to my past jobs and habits, you can surely tell I was so indecisive and was lost.

Luckily, the agency had an opportunity anticipating me. I had optimistic thoughts in my head that this was the right path for me. They hooked me up with a job in a warehouse. With the support of a job coach by my side and to watch over me, I felt more comfortable at work.

Of course, I still had major anxiety and social anxiety on the job, but I have come far enough to where I just be myself. I also have gotten comfortable to not worry about what people say or think. I am there to work. The nice thing about it is that it keeps me busy on my feet and it's repetitive.

It was a sense of relief that there was no customer contact. This job was a fit. Whenever I'd stress or have deep thoughts, my mind would give me faith that I wouldn't be there forever, and that I was just there to gain experience and be able to move on after. I found doing something with my hands especially helpful in not getting so distracted. My job coach's presence gave me a sense of confidence and helped me get over my fears. Whenever stress would hit me during this job, I'd tell myself the phrase "If it isn't broken, don't fix it."

"In the End"

~

Linkin Park

My life was a roller coaster going through what I have with my brain trauma. I have met inspirational and generous people who have given me courage to never give up. Those are the kinds of people that I wanted to have in my life. Anxiety was a motivational stepper along the way. When I would see or meet other people with social anxiety, I could totally relate to them and understand how it feels. I would not judge them by any means.

After many tries of doing this alone, there were hints that I was getting nowhere without communication. Ironically, out of fear and anxiety, I pushed myself to reach out for help when it was needed. Sometimes if I just took action right away without overthinking, it would give me a sense of accomplishment. It was amazing to see how much things have changed when I put myself out there a little more and fought my anxiety out. At times, my adrenaline rushed like a race car and I'd have sweaty palms, but it meant that it was a challenge to grow.

One day when I was on my usual walk at the park,

I ran into this lady and her dog. They were on a walk just like me. Eventually we made a conversation, and we got to know each other. It was a pleasure to meet her and have her be a new friend to me. She was not pushy, but more like an encouraging, helpful motivational friend. Getting to know her, she motivated me in such positive ways to study hard, chase after whatever I want to do in life, and that doing what frightens me the most to get the most success in life. I had a listening ear and couldn't be happier with her drive. As we got to know each other on our daily walks, She'd tell me her life story when she was my age and that she could relate to all this usual anxiety, fear, college, bullies and the circle of young adult life.

After hearing it, I took her word for it and would use it as a guiding tool for myself. It really was a great guide to making big decisions in my twenties. We both had a hobby of hiking and would occasionally meet for long mile hikes. We didn't let the high, steep rocky hills stop us or stress us out — it was our friendship that made us finish and follow through. When I was explaining to my friend about my struggles in college and unable to keep up, she shook her head like that was a crazy reason to not continue. Her confidence gave to me that I should not give up. I bit the bullet and bravely started back to a community college and started fresh with some mediocre courses.

This was the Fall 2018 semester. My friend went with me to my counselor meeting to discuss classes and certificates beforehand, but I was skeptical and felt unsure about what I exactly wanted to do. I just went with my gut on health and psychology counseling. From previous times in college of getting frustrated and impatient with not understanding the directions, I've gotten over that negativity with these classes and developed a sense of patience, communication and self-worth. It was a dramatic change I went to from a couple years before when I tried out the business management courses. On occasion, I would get stuck on directions and such with my new classes but would reach out to the teachers and email them immediately with any questions, without worrying. My friend was a motivational inspiration to helping me with these useful techniques. Because of her, I have faced even more fears and come a long way.

As I grew up and got over my anxiety just a bit, I have gotten braver to stand up for myself. This anxiety journey took many mountains of stomach pains, high stress, worrying to get to where I am. I still have high social anxiety and stress all of the time. Each day, I'd practice and practice more ways to just embrace my anxiety and not take it so seriously. Whenever I'd get stressed out badly, I'd tell myself, "My anxiety comes in handy." I have found it helpful to cope with my daily struggles and problems with writing and for the most part – exercising. Over time, I realized it helped me clear my head in a peaceful way. Was it easy to grow out of my shell? No it was not an easy journey. It is who I am and my style.

All along, I was an introvert. I am not a people

hater, just seemed to find joy in doing activities by myself. It was when I was in my early twenties that I liked making small talk with people and would just be myself. I didn't feel judged or feel insecure as much when I'd be eyeballed. I have grown to the point of knowing what kind's of things I like to do, types of people I like to click with, and have gotten a better glimpse of my lifestyle. I've been dealing with indecisiveness for many years. I would take forever to make decisions whether it would be what to major in, what kind of work I'd like to do, where to eat, and the list goes on.

My social anxiety and learning disability will follow me on this journey for a really long time, but I am happy with that. At times, I might hyperventilate and kill my brain to take a chance at saying something. I have climbed mountains to get this far. I am different then most people my age.

I have been doing my best to start over and get into the habit of making good decisions to become an adult.

I felt sad and ashamed when other students my age would be off to college and then graduated. I tried to feel happy enough that I graduated high school before them.

Through experience and practice, I would work on telling them that it just wasn't the path for me. The truth is living with social anxiety and having a learning disability has held me back from it. As my defeats were growing, I was starting realize over time to not go with just one option, but to keep all options open and compare them.

I had to be mentally prepared and set my mind to it. Instead of saying "I can't," which haunted me all through elementary, middle and high school, I would convince myself to focus more on "I can." Negativity would do nothing but just use of time in an unhealthy way. I was not alone in this though. It was with help of inspirational, amazing people who helped me move forward and make realistic decisions.

No matter the failures or hardships, my friend showed me that the only way I would get over my fears were to FACE it. As the years have gone by, I fought to prove and show others what I can do. I will not let my past define me. All I can do is move forward and embrace who I am and control my destiny.

But in the end, what matters is what I make of myself in this life. I used to think that time was super slow and didn't move at all, but it sure has gone by super fast.

Without all of that trauma I went through, I wouldn't of been this wise and strong. Anxiety, I found, to be a great helper and supporter to me. Even though it has thrown roadblocks at me, it was also like a driven force that helped me grow and face challenges that I went through all along the years growing up. Having social anxiety or being shy doesn't necessarily mean you are snooty, stuck up or conceited. As a person who has been through this, I can understand when others go through this and am not one to judge. No matter the hardships or amount of fear you have, there is always something creative and amazing one can offer. I still have a lot of improvements to make on myself, both internally and externally, especially my anxiety.

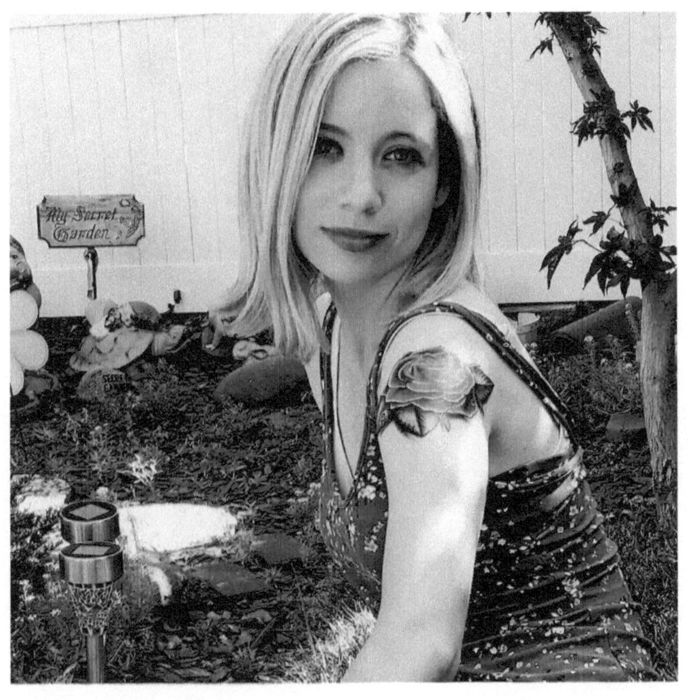

SIERRA CRISLIP is the survivor of a rare brain trauma, Hypothalamic Hamartoma. Despite it, she's gone on to graduate from high school early and obtained employment with the help of a job coach. "Even though you can't see my disability," Sierra says, "I want to put the word out there and help others going through the same thing." Her HH story is on the Hope For Hypothalamic Hamartoma's website. She resides in California.

www.ingramcontent.com/pod-product-compliance
Lightning Source LLC
Chambersburg PA
CBHW051227250726
48655CB00006B/2635